ACHIEVE YOUR WEIGHT LOSS RESOLUTIONS

Keeping Your Weight Loss Resolutions for the New Year

Copyright

The information provided herein is stated to be truthful and consistent, in that any liability, in terms of inattention or otherwise, by any usage or abuse of any policies, processes, or directions contained within is the solitary and utter responsibility of the recipient reader. Under no circumstances will any legal responsibility or blame be held against the publisher for any reparation, damages, or monetary loss due to the information herein, either directly or indirectly.

Respective authors own all copyrights not held by the publisher.

The information herein is offered for informational purposes solely, and is universal as so. The presentation of the information is without contract or any type of guarantee assurance.

The trademarks that are used are without any consent, and the publication of the trademark is without permission or backing by the trademark owner. All trademarks and brands within this book are for clarifying purposes only and are the owned by the owners themselves, not affiliated with this document.

Introduction

With the New Year fast approaching, it is about time you got the fitness that you so desperately desire. There's a consensus that thin is way better than fat. So people often strive to achieve exceptional leanness in a bid to not only look attractive, but to also help improve their quality of life, enhance their overall health, and regain some sense of control over their appearance. Sometimes, we realize too late that our weight impedes our lifestyle or outward appeal. Other times, it gets to the point that it begins to impact negatively on our health. Overweight people are at the risk of developing potentially life-threatening illnesses such as cancers or type 2 diabetes. Also, there's the risk of ending up with a heart disease, sleep apnea, gallstones, or high blood pressure.

Overweight often leads to undesirable outcomes for individuals. Some get to experience shame and embarrassment both from peers and colleagues who see the break of every dawn as an opportunity to ridicule their "fat" friends. Such encounters often cause people to experience low self-esteem.

It gets so worse that others become depressed and start to doubt themselves. With doubts slowly creeping in, their ability to get ahead in their career gets impeded. The cost of gaining so much weight can be too much to bear for anyone regardless of their age or gender, race or complexion. Most times, the motivation to avoid or reverse these conditions is what leads people to seek a solution to their weight problems.

If that sounds like you, then this book offers an opportunity for you to overcome your situation and take back control of how your body looks and is perceived by others. It provides you the chance to rebuild your image, build and maintain a good relationship, as well as feel optimistic about your life. Read on to find out more about how you can be in charge of your life.

9 steps to achieve your fitness goal

<u>Listing your goals</u>

In this step, you are to list everything you could think of that will help you achieve those goals. Did you notice the use of 'everything,' just name them here. The more understandable your list is, the more motivated you will become to achieve them. Don't complicate your goals no matter how long there are. The more intense your desire towards your goal is, the more you will believe the possibility of achieving them. So be committed towards them.

<u>Know your long-term goals</u>

Think about your health, your fitness, the future and what you want to accomplish in the long run. Maybe you want to lose 50 pounds in the New Year. Then put it down in writing, place it where you will always see this vision every morning and as you are about to sleep. Next, you have to hold yourself responsible and accountable for that goal and make a firm determination to pursue this goal with all your strength and mind, doing one thing at a time. Putting it down on paper and placing it where it will always be visible to you is like creating a covenant you have to stick to. Place that paper on your bedroom war or mirror— just in a place, you will be able to look on a daily basis. This will serve as a constant reminder of the pact you made with yourself to reach your goal as the year progresses. With this in place, you will be amazed at the result. Before March, you should be seeing some little goals achieved and just like the last point says, reward yourself and keep moving.

Set Short-term goals

Writing your long-term goals is a great beginning, achieving them requires scaling some steps to help get you achieve it smoothly. After all, we all know that losing 50 pounds doesn't just happen simply because you wrote it down. It happens because you are determined to lose that weight. For instance, you can create monthly goals, weekly or daily goals. An example of a weekly goal is to lose 1-2 pounds per week in a very healthy way. Statistics reveal that 97% of people who do not write their goals down didn't achieve those goals. Unwritten goals are very hard if not impossible to achieve. You can easily forget an unwritten goal, or some other goals may override them. Go ahead and create a monthly goal of losing 4-5 pounds in a month.

Make your goals measurable

Measurable goals are easily attained. Breaking goals down into an attainable level is a faster and most recommended way of achieving goals. How do you know you are making progress if you have no way of tracking your progress? Thus, you must set a key performance indicator, or a success indicator to help you measure when you are achieving goals. How will you know you're on the right path if there is no measuring scale? You can easily measure your weight because there is a weighing balance. The lesson here is to ensure your goals must be scalable and measurable. Doing weekly or monthly weigh-ins ensure you are on track with both your short-term and long-term goals.

Make a Plan

Put your goals into the plan, i.e., strategize on those goals. Take your list, organize, and put a 'verb' it into the plan. If there are long, attach the time factor in them, it will help you to organize them. And learn to organize in the order of priority and importance to you.

Make time-bound goals

Be time-bound, work with a deadline in view.

Setting deadlines act as a "tracking system" on your subconscious mind and begin to move you faster toward your goal while at the same time moving your goals towards you. A goal deadline helps you to know when that goal is due and when you need to move to the next goal. You may attain your goal before the deadline, when you do that, reward yourself. But if you don't set a deadline you will just be going toward your goals blindly and welcoming anything that comes your way.

<u>*Find Motivation*</u>

We have been using SMART goals model to help you achieve your fitness goal. From what has been considered thus far, it is clear that some goals are more likely to be achieved than others. The major cause of this is called intrinsic motivation. Intrinsic motivation is asking yourself if your long-term goal is something you want or is it what you want to achieve for someone else. Do you want to get fit just to be attracted to the opposite sex or you want to get fit for healthy living?

The implication is that if you're working toward achieving a goal for any other reason than yourself, you're far less likely to succeed in that goal. It's a simple law. Trying to please people or look good for peoples admiration is a goal you won't achieve or rather a goal you will lose faith on very soon. Thus, avoid setting goals if your interest and mind aren't into it.

Reward yourself

You must realize that the process of getting fit or losing weight is a journey, perhaps a long one indeed. If you drudge through will make your days miserable because fitness results do not come as fast as expected, hence making you hate every activity you are doing. Find activities you enjoy, one you have the passion for, and that will help you reach your short- and long-term goals. Remember, any short-term goal that is achieved is a deliverable of the long-term goal, and as such, you should reward yourself. You can take yourself to the cinema, or go to that museum as a way of rewarding yourself.

Rewarding yourself can also be buying yourself a gift. Achieving a short-term goal is enough reason to get yourself that gift you have wanted to have. Learn to reward yourself.

Take the first step

Take action. After all said and done, more is said than done. This is the biggest enemy of achieving goals that many people have. Even after setting specific and smart goals, must have written them down and have organized their goals, the next thing to do is to take action. Start small but make sure you are doing something. Don't procrastinate. Just do something.

Chapter One

Exercise and Fitness

The importance of exercise in helping to maintain weight loss or prevent excess weight gain cannot be over-emphasized. You burn calories when you engage in physical activity. As such, the more intense the activity you participate in, the more calories your burn. Beyond just burning calories, exercise is essential to your quest for fitness. It benefits you in ways such as:

Exercise helps to boost energy. Regular exercising helps to improve muscle strength and raise endurance. It supplies power and nutrients to body tissues and supports the cardiovascular system to work more efficiently. With an improvement in heart and lung health comes more energy.

Exercise helps to improve mood. Exercise helps provide emotional lift by stimulating various brain chemicals that can induce excitement and relaxation. Exercise helps you to sleep better, boosting your mental health as a result. Also, engaging in regular exercising will make you feel better about your outward appearance, which will, in turn, boost your confidence and enhance your self-esteem.

Exercise helps combat health conditions and diseases. Exercise helps you to fight and manage a broad range of health problems such as type 2 diabetes, stroke, metabolic syndrome, arthritis, and certain types of cancers, among others.

Effective Exercises That Help with Weight Loss

An exercise is a useful tool for a weight loss journey. However, you should know that training alone will not suffice if you are looking to lose weight fast. A successful weight loss ensues when you effectively combine exercise, proper eating, and healthy lifestyle habits. Also, it is essential to note that weight loss plans work differently for different people. What worked for Mr. A might not work for Mr. B.

With that being said, some exercises and workouts are helpful to your weight loss efforts. They help you to lose weight and change your body composition in a way that would make you feel proud of yourself. Typically, high-intensity exercises and workouts work best for weight loss, as they help to burn plenty of calories within a short period. Make them a part of your routine and watch how much change they would make in your outward appearance. To see results, however, it is essential to bear in mind that you will need to push yourself to the limits during every workout. Also, it is recommended that you find an exercise you enjoy to make it more fun and engaging. The following drills will help benefit your weight loss endeavor.

Interval Training: This is a training technique where participants alternate periods of quick, intense bursts of exercise with short, and seldom active recovery periods. This type of activity helps to keep the participant's heart rate elevated, increase fitness and allows them to burn calories in a short amount of time. One of such exercises is a cardio blaster, which requires you to use several muscles in your body including hamstrings, quads, core, and glutes.

The idea is that the more muscles you utilize; the more calories you are going to burn because all muscles incorporated require energy to work. Also, the more energy you use, the higher your calories will burn. It helps to enhance fitness levels and burn plenty of calories within a short time.

How to Do It:

You should first warm up for about 15 minutes. Next, bike, run, or row for 3 minutes at 90- and 95% of your maximum heart rate. If you're using a scale of 1 – 10, it should translate to about 8.5 or 9. After that, take approximately 3 minutes' active recover, and then conclude with a 10-minute cooldown. This kind of training not only help you to lose weight but also strengthens your cardiovascular system, improving your overall health.

Weight Training: Weight training is one of the most regular workouts that aids weight loss. This is because weight training has been shown to increase a participant's resting metabolic rate. What this means is that whoever lifts a weight, for instance, will continue to burn calories even after they have finished working out. This occurrence is known as the afterburn effect. Adding weight training to your routine at least three times a week you keep your body in shape and working correctly. To do this, do one set of the training in order and do not rest in between. Repeat the entire circuit three more times (four times in total). It is recommended to do this for up to thirty minutes of total time.

How to Do It:

Firstly, you do a plie punch by holding a pair of dumbbells at hips level with your elbows behind your body. Keep a standing position with your heels together, then turn your toes out about 45 degrees. Press your heels together and hold position, then extend your left arm in front of your shoulder and keep your palm facing down.

Secondly, you take a wide step to your right and switch arms, press your right arm forward as your left elbow bends, lower into a grand plie position by bending both knees out over your toes, with your shoulders stacked over your hips. Next, slide your right heel back into left as you switch arms. That completes one rep. Repeat ten times, and remember to alternate sides each time.

After completing the plie punch, you **thrust and throw.** To begin, assume a squat position and hinge about 45 degrees forward from your hips, reach the dumbbells to the floor and bend your elbow and weights to either side of your body. Squeeze your shoulder blades down and hold together.

Next, squat down to the floor and stretch out your arms, press the dumbbells into the ground directly below your shoulders. Then jump feet back to take a full plank position, draw your abs in tight, then jump feet back in and go back to your starting position. Like plie punch, this also requires four sets and ten reps.

Up next is **Spiderman pushups**. You begin this exercise by assuming a full plank position and placing your hands marginally wider. Keep your feet together. Next, lower into a pushup. Lift your left knee into your left arm (you can tap your knee to elbow, if possible). Return to the beginning and repeat, alternating your legs on each rep. Make 10 reps in total and a maximum of 4 sets.

Another effective workout is the **skull crush crunch**. To begin, grab a pair of dumbbells and lie faceup with your knees and hips bent about 90 degrees. Also, turn your elbows about 90 degrees such that the weights are in line with your shoulders. Keep your palms facing in.

Next, brace your abs in tight and crunch up. Lift your head and shoulders off the floor as your arms extend to the ceiling (keep your elbows lined up over your shoulders). Slowly start again and repeat. Do 4 sets and 15 reps.

Lastly, you can do a **hovering lunge and side tap**. To do this, grab a dumbbell in your left hand and assume a lunge position (ensure to bring back your knee not more than a few inches above the floor), place your left leg forward and extend your right arm up by your ear. Keep your left arm down by the side.

Next, you brace your abs in tight and bend at your waist. Reach your left hand to the floor, then tap the end of the dumbbell to the ground, look up to your right hand. That's it. Start all over again and repeat. Do all 15 reps on the first side, then repeat on the other side to complete a set. You will need to complete 4 sets in all.

Boot Camp: Boot camp is an excellent workout technique the ensures fitness by keeping your metabolism elevated all day. The exercise combines interval and resistance styles of training, allowing you to perform some tasks where some are more cardio-focused, while others are strength-centric, all-out for short bursts of time. Brief periods of rest accompany these. For those who are doing this for the first time, it is advisable to speak to an instructor, so that they can help you determine when you need to take it up a notch. It is recommended that newbies begin slowly, to allow their body to adapt to the training technique gradually. With time, you can start to crank it up. Just remember not to be too hard on yourself.

As mentioned above, boot camp-style training gets results fast by combining heart-rate revving cardio moves with multi-joint strength exercises to enable you to burn plenty of calories and tone every inch of your body. So, if you wish to undertake these exercises at home and save some cash, you can prepare a workout space outside your home or indoors. To do this, arrange five stations in a large circle in your workout area. Then mark each position with a label or mark them in your head. Next, put a jump rope at the first station, place a medicine ball at the second, and two cones measured at about four feet apart at the third. Place a pair of dumbbells at the fourth station and leave the fifth position open to complete the marking.

The workout is split into three circuits of five exercises each. Perform each exercise for one minute in order and do not rest between stations. Execute two rounds of the first circuit (slides two through six), then rest for one to two minutes and move on to the second circuit (slides seven through eleven). Continue the pattern until you have done two rounds of all three courses. This should take you a total time of up to one hour.

<h3 style="text-align:center">Other Exercises for effective weight loss:</h3>

Jump Rope: this is a fundamental step that requires you to jump rope as frequently and as swiftly as you can. Do two sets and keep the reps at one minute.

Medicine Ball Strength Exercise: to do this exercise, take a pushup position with the ball under one of your hands. Do a pushup, and as your arms extend, roll the ball to the other side. Do another pushup. This time, hold the ball firmly under the opposite arm. Get on with it, alternating both hands. Do two sets and keep the reps at one minute.

Cone Cardio Drill: for starters, stand in the middle of the two cones you placed earlier, with one in the front and the other behind your body. Quickly start to jog in a figure 8 style by making a circle around the front cone. Then run back to circle the back cone. Ensure to keep your body always facing forward. As with the rest, do two sets and keep the reps at one minute.

Deadlift Row: doing this exercise requires you to stand with your feet hip-width apart, and your knees slightly bent. Engage your abs and hold the dumbbells, then hinge forward, bringing your chest toward the floor. Keep your spine naturally straight.

Next, bend your elbows and pull the dumbbells to sides of your torso, squeeze your shoulder blades back together, then extend your arms to return to the starting position. Do two sets and a minute reps.

Bodyweight Cardio Drill: this high knees technique requires you to run in place with your hands in front of your body. Keep your palms facing down. Try to tap your knees to your palms as your legs alternate quickly. Do two sets and one-minute reps.

Jump Rope: this is a crossover jump technique where you try to cross your arms in front of your body while the rope is in the air. Do two sets and a minute reps.

Medicine Ball Strength: this is a squat chops technique. To do it, stand with your feet wide and hold the medicine ball overhead.

Next, quickly lower into a deep squat position, then chop the ball down to the ground. Get back to the position from where you started and repeat the process. For more intensity, you can add a jump during the chop. As usual, do two sets and 1-minute reps.

Cone Cardio Drill: this is a side shuffle touchdown procedure. To perform it, stand in between two cones placed at about four feet apart. Then quickly shuffle to the right. After that, tap the cone.

Shuffle to the immediately after and tap the other cone. Repeat the technique as quickly as possible. Do two sets and 1-minute reps.

Dumbbell Strength Exercise: this exercise technique involves rear lunge and curl. Firstly, grab a pair of dumbbells and stand with your feet together. Keep your knees slightly bent, then bend your elbows by the sides. Keep your palms facing up.

Secondly, step your right leg back and lower into a lunge position. Bend both knees at 90 degrees as you extend your arms down by the sides. Then curl your arms up as you revert to the starting position. Repeat the process on the opposite side. Keep on alternating your legs until you complete the set. Perform two sets and a minute reps.

Bodyweight Cardio Drill: to do these burpees exercise technique, squat down to the floor and place your hands below your shoulders, then quickly jump feet back into a plank position.

Next, jump feet back into a squat position and then forcibly jump up. Reaching your arms overhead. For more challenge, you can add a pushup. Perform two sets and 1-minute reps.

Jump Rope: this is a boxer's jump technique. To do it, alternate tapping your heels slightly in front of your body while landing. Do two sets and a minute rep.

Medicine Ball Strength: this is a crunch and catch technique. To execute, lie faceup with your knees bent and your feet flat. Hold the ball in in front of your chest. Sit up quickly and toss the ball up in the air. Catch it and roll down through your spine with your abs tight and revert to the beginning. Do two sets and 1-minute reps.

Cone Cardio Drill: this is a plank walk exercise procedure. Start in a plank position to the right side of one of the cones. Then lift your right hand and reach across your body to tap the cone.

Next, walk with your hands and feet out to the right until you are close to the opposite cone. Tap the cone with your left hand. Redo the exercise as quickly as possible and keep your abs tight so that your lower back does not sag. Do two sets and 1-minute reps.

Dumbbell Strength Exercise: this is a squat to press technique. To do, hold the dumbbells in front of your shoulders with your palms facing in. Then lower into a shallow squat so that you can gain power.

Next, extend your legs as your arms press overhead. Then move as fast as possible. Do two sets and a minute reps.

Body Cardio Drill: this involves a mountain climbers' technique. Assume a full plank position and alternate bending one of your knees into your chest as quickly as possible. Do two sets and a minute reps.

Chapter Two

Healthy Eating and Nutrition

Weight loss is best achieved through a combination of proper diet and exercise. When followed correctly, healthy eating and nutrition will enable you to reap so many benefits in a short amount of time. Adkins diet and other similar weight loss diet plans have helped popularized the low-carb, real-food based menu that allows you to eat healthily, lose weight, and feel great every day. A low-carb diet is a diet type that limits carbohydrates such as those found in starchy vegetables, sugary foods, grains, and fruit. Instead, it encourages the consumption of foods that are high in protein and healthy fat. Various studies show that these types of diet can cause weight loss and help improve overall health.

They aid weight loss by reducing hunger and enhance body health by controlling insulin and blood sugar, reducing the risk for certain types of cancer, and lowering the risk for heart diseases factors. Also, low-carb diets help to enhance cognitive performance, among other things.

However, you should bear in mind that what you should eat depends on how much exercise you do and how much weight you have to lose. Ensure to eat the right amount of food that makes you feel better. To see changes fast, you should consider low-carb, real diet as a way of eating, a lifestyle. Embrace it and see how much difference it will make in your body composition. As such, we take you through the foods you should eat and those you should avoid

<u>**Best Foods You Are Not Eating**</u>

If you are the type of person that avoids natural, unprocessed foods, then you must make a diet change if you are looking to lose weight and lead a healthy lifestyle. Natural and unprocessed foods are a secret weapon for individuals who have unsuccessfully tried to torch calories. Consequently, here are some healthy foods you should eat:

Fish: fish is rich in omega-3 fatty acids, which are crucial for your health. Omega-3 fatty acids help to improve outward appearance, especially skin health, boosts body immunity, improve your mood, prevent depression, and improves cardiovascular health. Also, they balance cholesterol levels, stabilize blood sugar levels and help to prevent diabetes, among others. Fish such as salmon, cod, sardines, trout, tuna, haddock, and many others contribute to complementing your weight loss efforts. Weight caught fish works best.

Meat: Unprocessed meat is right for you if you are looking to lose weight and maintain fitness. Unprocessed meat is excellent for you, especially if the animals were fed natural foods, such as beef from grass-fed cows. Beef, lamb, pork, chicken, etc. work well. However, lean meat and chicken breast are the best of the lot.

Bananas:

Like apples, bananas are also rich in potassium and contain multivitamins which are essential for weight loss. They are filling and help you to resist the cravings for fast food and other junk foods. Moreover, banana boosts the metabolic rate, thereby melting the body fat. Include this in your diet today, and your body weight becomes a history.

Whole Eggs: Eggs are some of the most nutritious foods you can consume if you need to lose weight. They are high in protein, contain healthy fat, and help make you full with a meager amount of calories. Also, eggs are abundantly nutrient dense. As such, they help provide you with all the nutrients you need. Almost all the nutrients you need on a calorie restricted diet are found in egg yolks, as it is the most nutritious and healthiest part of whole eggs.

Vegetables: leafy greens like spinach, kale, collards, Swiss chards, among others have various properties that make them ideal for a weight loss diet. Greens are low in both carbohydrates and calories but contain high amounts of fiber. They allow you to increase the volume of your meals without risking an increase in the number of calories. Leafy greens are highly nutritious and contain various types of essential vitamins, minerals, and antioxidants that the body needs, such as calcium, which itself has been shown to help in burning fats.

On their part, cruciferous vegetables such as broccoli, cabbage, cauliflower, and Brussels sprouts help with weight loss. Like leafy greens, they contain high amounts of fiber and can be incredibly fulfilling. In addition, they contain reasonable amounts of protein that help keep you in good health. They combine fiber, protein, as well as low energy density, all of which help with weight loss.

Fruit: fruits such as avocado are loaded with healthy fats. Avocados are exceptionally rich in monounsaturated oleic acid, which is the same type of acid found in olive oil. They lower blood pressure and increase fat burning to help with your weight loss endeavors. Also, they prevent type 2 diabetes and protect body cells from radical damage. Avocados also contain many essential nutrients such as fiber and potassium.

Similarly, Grapefruit has shown great potential when it comes to weight loss. Various studies show that eating fresh grapefruit before meals cause weight loss. Also, grapefruit has been found to help with the reduction of insulin resistance.

In the same vein, fruits like oranges, mangoes, etc. contain properties that make them weight loss friendly. Nonetheless, if you have some intolerance to fructose or you are on a very low carb, it is advisable to minimize fruit consumption. As always, though, it is important to eat in moderation.

<u>*Nuts and Seeds:*</u> nuts contain balanced amounts of fiber, protein, and healthy fats that help cause weight loss and improve metabolic health. Various studies have shown that individuals who eat nuts tend to be leaner and healthier than those who don't. Also, seeds such as chia seeds are low carb friendly and one of the best sources of fiber you can find around. Their high fiber content means that they can absorb between 11 to 12 times their weight in water. This means that they expand in your stomach and make you feel full for a very long time. Therefore, whether it is walnuts, almonds, or sunflower seeds, you should endeavor to eat them if you are looking to lose weight. However, you should do so in moderation.

Potatoes: White, boiled potatoes have many properties that make them the perfect food not only for those who seek to lose weight but also for people who desire optimal health. They contain an impressively broad range of nutrients, providing you with almost everything you need. Potatoes contain a high volume of potassium, which helps so much with blood pressure control. They aid weight loss by making you feel naturally full for long spells, causing you to eat less of other foods. When allowed to cool down after being boiled, white potatoes usually form significant quantities of resistant starch. The fiber-like substance has been shown to have lots of health benefits including promoting weight loss.

Fats and oils: oils such as coconut oil is rich in fatty acids referred to as Medium Chain Triglycerides (MCTs). These fatty acids contain properties that enable them to improve satiety. So, make it a point to replace some of your other cooking fats with not just coconut oil but extra virgin olive oil, lard, butter, etc.

Liquids That Promote Weight Loss

The following drinks will help improve your weight loss endeavors:

Tea: Tea contains high amounts of antioxidants that are healthy and help with weight loss. Also, tea contains less caffeine than coffee. So, individuals who are sensitive to coffee can consume tea instead.

Green Tea:

Green tea works as a body detoxifier, which helps in burning the excess body fat in the body. Consuming green tea daily can make your skin glow, as well as, make your tummy flat plus other additional benefits you can get from this drink. Do you have one already? If no, then get it before today ends.

Coffee: coffee is a healthy drink that is very rich in antioxidants. This makes it useful for heart health and other illnesses.

Water: as water is 100% calorie-free, it can be beneficial to weight loss. Water is said to help torch calories and even suppress appetite when consumed before meals. More so, replacing beverages with water will see you cut back on sugar, which can adversely affect your weight loss efforts.

<u>**How to take water to promote weight loss**</u>

Every day take 150cl of bottle water as early as 6 A.M, This must not be a pet can water, it can just be a glass of water, the objective it just to get the amount of water to take accurately. Take it before and after meal and about what has been said above

Once it is 1:00 P.M before you go for lunch, you should also get a 75cl sized water, turn it into a cup and gulp it all, don't remain for anyone.

Also, around 5:00 P.M before your dinner, you are to turn another 75cl of water into another cup again and finish it once.

If you consistently do this for long, you should expect to be happy with your health status. Though it will be stressful at first but with time, you will get used to this daily diet, and it will become a normal thing for you. Sometimes you might feel dizzy or weak after drinking water, but trust me, this is the best therapy you can give to yourself. The benefits you should look out for as you regularly take this diet include a balanced your lymph system which helps you perform your daily function efficiently and effectively and also help to balance your body fluids, diseases, and fight body infections. Also taking a good amount of water helps to purge toxins from the body, and this will result in keeping your skin glowing, clear, and attractive. Taking at least half liter of water every morning will help boost your body metabolism and lead to weight loss. Many do not know that drinking water on an empty stomach early in the morning purifies the colon thereby making it easier to absorb nutrients when taken, therefore what stops you from taking water regularly.

Lime Water

Aside the benefits obtained from taking lemon water, another supplement which has proven very effective and affordable is the lime water. Limes as we know it contains lots of vitamins, minerals, enzymes and phytonutrients which is highly needed in the body. The major difference is that Lemons happen to have just a little bit more fructose content, which only implies that it's more appealing to taste and its aroma also. Hence it is not surprising the health benefits this brings. Remember, more of words does nothing, it's only action that speaks louder than voice, therefore you should not just read but begin to practice what you read. Lime water is one of the best and cheapest ways to detoxify your body and burn stubborn fat within a very short period. The benefit of this lime water cannot be overemphasized as Lime water not only activate the liver and kidney to remove the excess body hormones (which includes estrogen and insulin) associated with increased production of fatty cells within the body. It also helps to stimulate bile production which in turn helps break down fat in the body system and rids them off as wastes.

Foods to Avoid During Weight Loss

You should limit your consumption of or avoid the following foods altogether if you are looking to lose weight:

Sugar: added sugar is fattening and one of the chief causes of diseases such as diabetes, obesity, and cardiovascular disease.

Seed and Vegetable Oils: avoid eating processed fats that contain high amounts of omega-6 fatty acids. Omega-6 fatty acids are harmful when consumed in excess amounts. As such, you would do well to avoid oils such as corn oil, soybean oil, and others.

Grains: some grains can harm your weight loss attempts. Such grains contain gluten, which can be harmful to your body due to the vast range of complications it can cause. For this reason, you should avoid or consume grains like rye, barley, wheat, spelt, etc. in moderation. Instead, you should consume healthier whole grains like brown rice, oats, and quinoa, among others.

Trans Fats: avoid chemically modified fats, as they are bad for health and will negate your weight loss efforts. These type of fats are found in processed foods.

Highly Processed Foods: highly processed foods usually contain low nutrients and high unhealthy as well as unnatural chemicals.

Artificial Sweeteners: artificial sweeteners can cause obesity and other related diseases. Avoid sweeteners if you must stay fit. However, you can choose stevia if you badly need sweeteners.

Side Note:

* You can take soda without artificial sweeteners.

* Simple Rule: avoid calories.

* You can consume dark chocolate and alcohol in moderation. Dark chocolate contains high amounts healthy fast and antioxidants that help with weight loss. If you must take alcohol, choose dry wines and drinks that do not contain added sugar or carbohydrates. These include whiskey, vodka, etc. Remember, however, that you must consume alcohol in moderation

Chapter Three

3 Ways to Lose Belly Fat and Tone Your Legs

When it comes to burning fats in specific parts of your body, it can be hard to know what to do. However, targeting belly fat is one of the ways you can stay lean and keep fit. With the end of year fast approaching, there's no better time to lose belly fat and tone your legs. You can firm up the areas of your body covered in a layer of fat and tone your legs through a combination of the following:

1. **Create a Calorie Deficit:** As you would already know by now, calories are bad news for weight loss. Being in a calorie deficit enables you to get rid of fat in any part of your body. It is essential to burn off more calories than you consume on a regular basis if you must lose that belly fat. To pull this off, you will need to lower your food intake and move around more. Make it a duty to eat nutrient-dense whole foods such as lean meats, quinoa, fish, and vegetables, among others.

2. **Perform some resistance training**. Resistance training helps to add a more toned look to your entire body muscles and make them look firm. In fact, lifting heavy weights help you to achieve fitness fast and ensure that develop that you develop a toned physique. You should look to train with a resistance that induces fatigue between 8-12 reps. The higher reps you can do, the better, but don't push yourself too hard, especially when you are just beginning. Also, it is essential to aim to do exercises that target every muscle group rather than just pounding your legs. Compound lifts like pull ups, press ups, deadlifts, and even lunges help to enhance overall calorie burn while increasing your total fat-free mass as well as you're your resting metabolic rate. Work your legs to fatigue with various exercises two to three times per week. Include as a part of your training plan and see how much change they will make to belly and leg composition.

The under listed exercises will help you shed belly fat and tone your leg muscles:

Squat Pause: Squat pause is a constant presence in any exercise regimen. That's because it works well when it comes to achieving fitness and toning your legs.

How to Do It:

a. Begin with your feet standing shoulder width apart. Keep your toes pointing toward eleven- and one o'clock.
b. Next, keep your chest proud and then lower down to assume a full squat position. Do this until your upper leg passes parallel to the ground.
c. When at the base, pause for between two to three seconds.
d. Drive up. But as you do so, ensure to push your knees out. To prevent your knees from collapsing inwards, imagine you're screwing your heels into the floor.
e. Squeeze your thighs and glutes at the top. Repeat between 10 to 12 times.

2. **Reverse Slide Lunges.** This training technique helps to stabilize your lower body while working your quads, glutes, as well as hamstrings.

How to Do It:

    a. Put a towel or slider underneath one of your foot, and make to stand up straight. Face forward.

    b. Slide back the towel using one foot and let your knee drop into a lunge position.

    c. Keep your chest proud, then drive up from the inactive leg back, thrust your hips forward, then get back up into a standing position.

    d. Squeeze both your thighs and glutes at the top. Redo the exercise 10 to 12 times on each leg.

    e. To add more resistance, you can hold a weight such as a kettlebell.

3. **Barbell Hip Thrust**. This is yet another lower body exercise that targets both belly fat and leg muscle toning. The technique engages tons of muscle mass in your glutes.

How to Do It:

- Place a bench and then assume a seating position with the chair directly behind you. Rest your shoulder blades on the bench.
- Grab a padded barbell and hold it over your hips, then bend your legs keeping your feet shoulder-width apart.
- Drive through your feet to start the movement, then extend your hips vertically, through the bar.
- Next, hold your feet flat on the ground, using the bench to support your weight.
- Squeeze glutes at the top. After that, slowly lower the bar back to the point where you started.

Chapter Four

Weight Loss Pills: Do They Work?

A lot of people often hail weight loss pills as the fastest and easiest way to slim down. But how safe are these pills and which ones work?

Well, the truth is that there are pills that have been found to aid weight loss. However, they are not as much of a quick fix as they are being touted to be. However, weight loss pills are an effective tool to aid weight loss when taken along with a fitness regime and diet. Weight loss pills work through one or more of the following mechanisms:

Promote fat burning. Some weight loss pills are designed to make you lose weight by making you burn a lot more calories.

Lower appetite. Certain weight loss drugs are intended to make you feel more full so that you eat less food, and consequently, fewer calories.

Reduce absorption. Some weight loss pills limit your body's ability to absorb fats, causing you to take in fewer calories.

With that out of the being said, here are some weight loss pills that are said to work:

Orlistat (Alli). This drug works by hindering the breakdown of fat in your gut, which will in turn, cause you to take in fewer calories from fat. Eleven different studies have been carried out on this pill so far. In those studies, it was found that the drug promotes weight loss by about six pounds of weight relative to a dummy pill. Also, the one research shows that the pill can reduce the risk of developing type 2 diabetes by about 37 percent. It has been shown to lower blood sugar slightly.

For all its benefits, however, Orlistat is said to have many digestive side effects. These consist of flatulence, loose and oily stools, frequent bowel movements, etc. Also, the drug may play a part in the deficiency of fat-soluble vitamins like vitamins A, D, E, as well as K.

Therefore, it is advisable to follow a low-fat diet while taking Alli, to minimize its side effects.

Meratrim. Meratrim is a weight loss pill that is said to make it harder for fat cells to multiply in the body. As a result, it lowers the amount of fat that they carry from the bloodstream and assists them in burning fat. A study carried out on 100 obese people who were placed on a strict 2000 calorie diet, alongside either Meratrim pill or a dummy pill shows that Meratrim is effective against weight loss. The study, which lasted for about eight weeks, saw the group placed on Meratrim drug loss 11 pounds of weight. This was in addition to them losing approximately 4.7 inches off their waistlines. In the same vein, Meratrim was also found to have a significant impact on the participants' quality of life, as it was found to reduce blood sugar levels, cholesterol, and triglycerides. Presently, no side effects have been reported about this pill.

Belviq. This drug works by curbing your appetite such that it makes you feel full. It is approved for long-term use. Also, the pill is sometimes used in the treatment of diabetes, high blood pressure, or high cholesterol. Belviq causes side effects like dizziness, headache, dry mouth, fatigue, constipation, and nausea. Its most common side effects in people with diabetes include low blood sugar, cough, back pain, headache, and cough.

Caution: Do not use Belviq if you are pregnant, as weight loss attempts during pregnancy can harm your baby.

Saxenda. This is an FDA-approved weight loss medication that helps with excess weight management as well as obesity. The pill mimics an intestinal hormone that signals to the brain that the stomach is full. Its side effects include vomiting, constipation, diarrhea, low blood pressure, nausea, as well as increased appetite. However, you should note that it can also cause serious side effects such as pancreatitis, kidney problems, raised heart rate, gallbladder disease, as well as suicidal thoughts.

Side Note:

*weight loss supplements like Garcina Cambogia Extract, Hydroxycut, caffeine, raspberry ketones, green coffee bean extract, glucomannan, green tea extract, etc. have also been found to aid weight in various scientific studies.

Chapter Five

Weight and Diabetes

Weight and diabetes usually affect each other. However, how they affect each other depends on circumstances, as you would see below.

Weight and Type 1 Diabetes

When an individual has type 1 diabetes, their body does not use glucose properly. As you may already know, glucose is sugar that serves as the primary source of energy for the body. Glucose levels in the body are regulated by a hormone known as insulin, which is formed in the pancreas. The pancreas fails to create enough insulin in people with type 1 diabetes. As such, untreated or undiagnosed type 1 diabetes can cause weight loss. This is because glucose gradually accumulates in the bloodstream if insulin is not available to move it to the muscles.

As glucose levels rise, the kidneys work to remove it through urine. This results in weight loss as a result of dehydration and depletion of calories from sugar that was not used as energy. Therefore, individuals with undetected or untreated type 1 diabetes often lose weight even if they have a usual or increased appetite. Nonetheless, their weight usually returns to normal once they are treated for type 1 diabetes.

While the occurrence of type 1 diabetes cannot be connected to being overweight, it is vital that you keep a healthy weight. Too much fat tissue in your body can impede the proper functioning of insulin. This could lead to higher insulin needs and difficulty controlling blood sugar.

Weight and Type 2 Diabetes

With type 2 diabetes, the pancreas still manufactures insulin, but the insulin does not work in the body as it should. This causes blood sugar levels to spike. Being overweight and obese increases people's risks for developing type 2 diabetes. This is especially true if a person has excess weight around their tummy. Therefore, being overweight and obese causes obesity in the following ways:

Inflammatory response. Various studies show that abdominal fat causes fat cells to discharge pro-inflammatory chemicals which can trigger the body to become less sensitive to the insulin it makes. This is because the pro-inflammatory chemicals disrupt the function of the cells that are responsive to insulin as well as their ability to respond to insulin. This scenario is usually referred to as insulin resistance, which is an indication of type 2 diabetes.

Disruption of fat metabolism. Excess weight gain is said to cause changes in the body's metabolism. In turn, such changes trigger fat tissue (known as adipose tissue) to discharge fat molecules into the bloodstream. This can affect insulin-responsive cells and bring about a reduction in insulin sensitivity.

As insulin sensitivity reduces, the pancreas can wear out from working too hard eventually. When this happens, the pancreas might be unable to produce enough insulin to keep blood glucose within a reasonable range. Type 2 diabetes results at this point.

To counteract this, you will need to embark on exercise and follow a strict diet to torch fat. For individuals with type 2 diabetes, exercising makes it easy to attain target blood sugar levels.

Chapter Six

The Paleo Diet

As far as achieving fitness goes, the paleo diet is one of the healthiest ways you can eat to stay lean, fit, and energetic. Sometimes called the caveman diet, Stone Age diet, primal diet, and hunter-gatherer diet, the paleo diet is a low-carb diet that is based on the diet of ancient humans. Consequently, it only permits the consumption of foods that are straight from the earth. These consist of fruits, vegetables, meats nuts, water, as well as seafood. The idea behind is that people should only eat foods that do not require technology to produce. The aim is to lower exposure to chemicals, pesticides, and antibiotics that didn't exist during the Paleolithic times. So basically, being on a paleo diet means giving up modern food. This means that you will have to avoid eating grains, added salt, dairy, or even legumes (such as beans, peanuts, lentils, and soybeans).

The philosophy behind the recent trend back to the Paleo nutrition is to keep things simple, by cutting out industrially processed foods and including fresh, naturally available food items we could grow around us. It is worthy of note that the Paleo diet is built around eating the way that we were meant to eat just like our parents did in time past before the advent of the technology age. Research revealed that they lived better than us regarding their health conditions. Fat diminishing system review is on the increase now, and one of its biggest selling points in the health domain is the claim that you can lose weight on the Paleo diet without even trying to get into any diminishing body routine. Yes, it is possible as, under the Paleo method, there is no calorie-measurement, punishing portion control, or intermittent fasts, yet fat reduction has been experienced by many who follow the Paleo diet meal.

The diet helps to reduce the body's glycemic load and enhance vitamin and nutrient consumption. Also, it contains an optimal balance of fat, protein, and carbohydrates, and has a healthy ratio of saturated-to-unsaturated fatty acids. Also, have it in mind that Paleo is not all food. Exercise forms a vital part of the paleo lifestyle. If you wish to survive in the stone age, as is the case with you going paleo, then you must understand that it is an on-the-go lifestyle that requires you to burn lots of calories on a daily basis.

While the demands of a paleo diet might seem easy to meet at first, it is essential to note that it is impossible to completely mimic our ancestors. Of the foods outlawed, certain ones can be consumed in moderation. Such exceptions mean that you can eat potatoes sparingly. Also, alcohol and honey are outlawed on the diet. But you can take red wine, as it is the closest option that you would find to a paleo drink. On its part, honey is far preferred to sugar or artificial sweeteners, if you must consume some sweets. Similarly, in spite of its strict restriction paleo diet exempts certain grains and dairy from the menu.

Summarily, here is a list of foods you can eat and does you should not:

Do Not Eat:

- Dairy
- Cereal grains
- Legumes
- Potatoes
- Refined sugar
- Processed foods

Eat:

- Fresh fruits
- Grass-fed meats
- Fresh vegetables
- Fish/seafood
- Nuts
- Eggs

Paleo Diet Meats: while all meats are allowed on the paleo diet, you should abstain from highly processed meats.

Chapter Seven

8 Dos and Don'ts of Weight Loss You Should Know

Whether it is exercise or a diet plan, following a weight loss plan is not an easy thing to do. So, these 8 tips will help you to understand how you can strike a balance that can help tone you up:

Do drink lots of water. Drinking lots of water help to lower calorie intake and reduce the risk of gaining weight, since water is naturally calorie-free. Also, drinking water will make you feel full, thereby reducing your consumption of other foods that contain calories. For a better result, substitute other beverages with water. Drinking a minimum of eight glasses of water a day will help keep you hydrated and rid your system of toxic waste substances.

Don't skip breakfast. Breakfast is arguably the most crucial meal of the day. Having breakfast enlivens and revives your system early enough to get you in top condition for the day. It kick-starts body metabolism and prevents you from getting hungrier later in the day. normally, people eat more during the day if they skip breakfast. Besides, studies have shown that individuals who eat breakfast lose weight faster than those who don't.

Do exercise. This point cannot be emphasized enough. The gym might not be your favorite spot. But if you are to lose weight, that has to change. You can make your house your own gym. Err, and, how about taking a walk? Regardless of how strict you follow a diet plan; you will end up achieving little weight loss if you fail to combine it with physical activity. Therefore, you could combine your diet plan (or pills) with walking for half an hour riding a bike, or go for a run. Just anything at all. It is important to keep working your body so you can get your heart pumping with a bit of cardio every 24 hours.

Do get a journal. Keeping a journal is important for your weight loss efforts. keeping a food journal will help you to keep track of the food you eat. When you keep a log of the food you consume, which foods are responsible for your body composition. A food journal enables you to see at a glance why your weight loss efforts are paying off – or not. Doing this will help you to control your calorie intake better.

Don't quit. Consistency builds success when it comes to weight loss. You should not let a lack of result in the immediate term discourage you from carrying on with your weight loss plan. If you are wondering why a certain diet or exercise isn't working for you like it did for your friend, remember that we all have different body types. What works for your friend might not work for you. However, calling it quits has never been the solution to any issue – nor will it ever be. Try other methods instead. It won't be too long before you find what works for you.

Do control the portion sizes in your meal. One of the secret ingredients of a successful weight loss plan is eating smaller portions of meals more often. Doing this helps to boost metabolism, which will, in turn, lead to weight loss.

Don't keep a single diet. The old clichéd saying, "variety is the spice of life" has never been apter than when it comes to weight loss. Vary your meals to make things more interesting. Keeping a single diet might cause you to lose interest. Once this happens, you will find yourself contemplating whether to quit the weight loss plan altogether. Experiment with new healthy foods to spice things up.

Don't deprive yourself of all treats. Don't be too hard on yourself; keep things interesting by consuming foods that you crave in moderation. Depending on the diet plan you are adopting, you do not have to create a forbidden foods list just because you are on a weight loss plan. Either that or you can replace those foods with lesser calorie alternatives.

Conclusion

Don't ever think of giving up your fitness goal. The world, society, and the environment will always give you the reason to give up. Whatever you want to achieve, the world will aid you. Be it the good or the bad; the society has a lot of things to aid in that decision of yours. But there is one that should be evergreen in your memory; never give up. There is this obvious truth that we all fail to admit, but we live with that truth which is the fact that none of us are inspired every day. We all have reason to give up because we are all exhausted

It is possible to achieve your weight loss goals when you battle weight loss with smart strategies. Remember, always aim to burn more calories than you eat. If the amount of calories that you consume is the same as the amount of energy that you burn, your weight will end up being the same. Eating fewer calories than you use up will cause your body to dig deep into its various fat reserves for the extra energy it needs. Weight loss then results

www.ingramcontent.com/pod-product-compliance
Lightning Source LLC
Chambersburg PA
CBHW050758240726
48654CB00008B/540